One, Two, What Do I Do?

A Children's Guide to Talking Back to OCD's Intrusive Thoughts

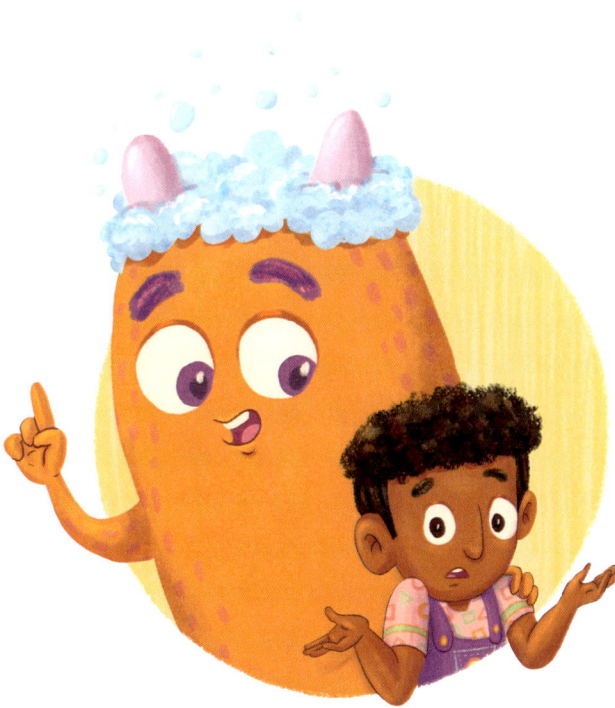

Megan Anne Barthle-Herrera, Ph.D.
Amanda Marie Balkhi, Ph.D.

Illustrated by
Yogita Chawdhary

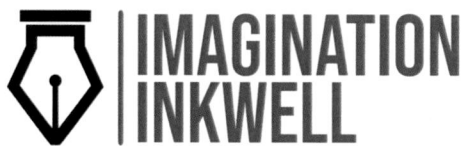

IMAGINATION INKWELL

ISBN-13: 979-8-218-27276-0

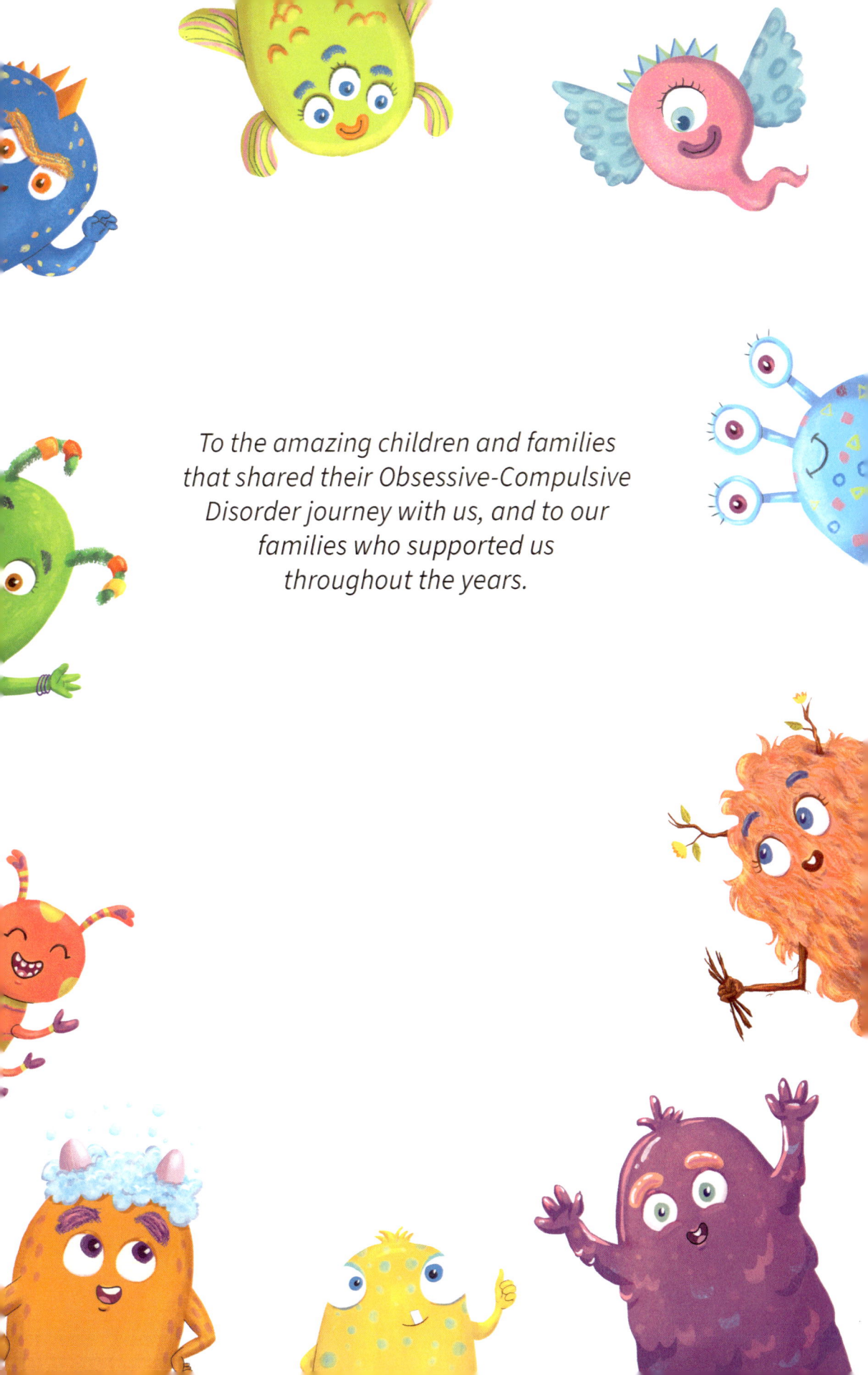

To the amazing children and families that shared their Obsessive-Compulsive Disorder journey with us, and to our families who supported us throughout the years.

We all have part of us that keeps us alert;
And shows us all the things that could make us hurt.

Like running in the street or climbing up too high,
Our brain tells us to be careful and what rules to apply.

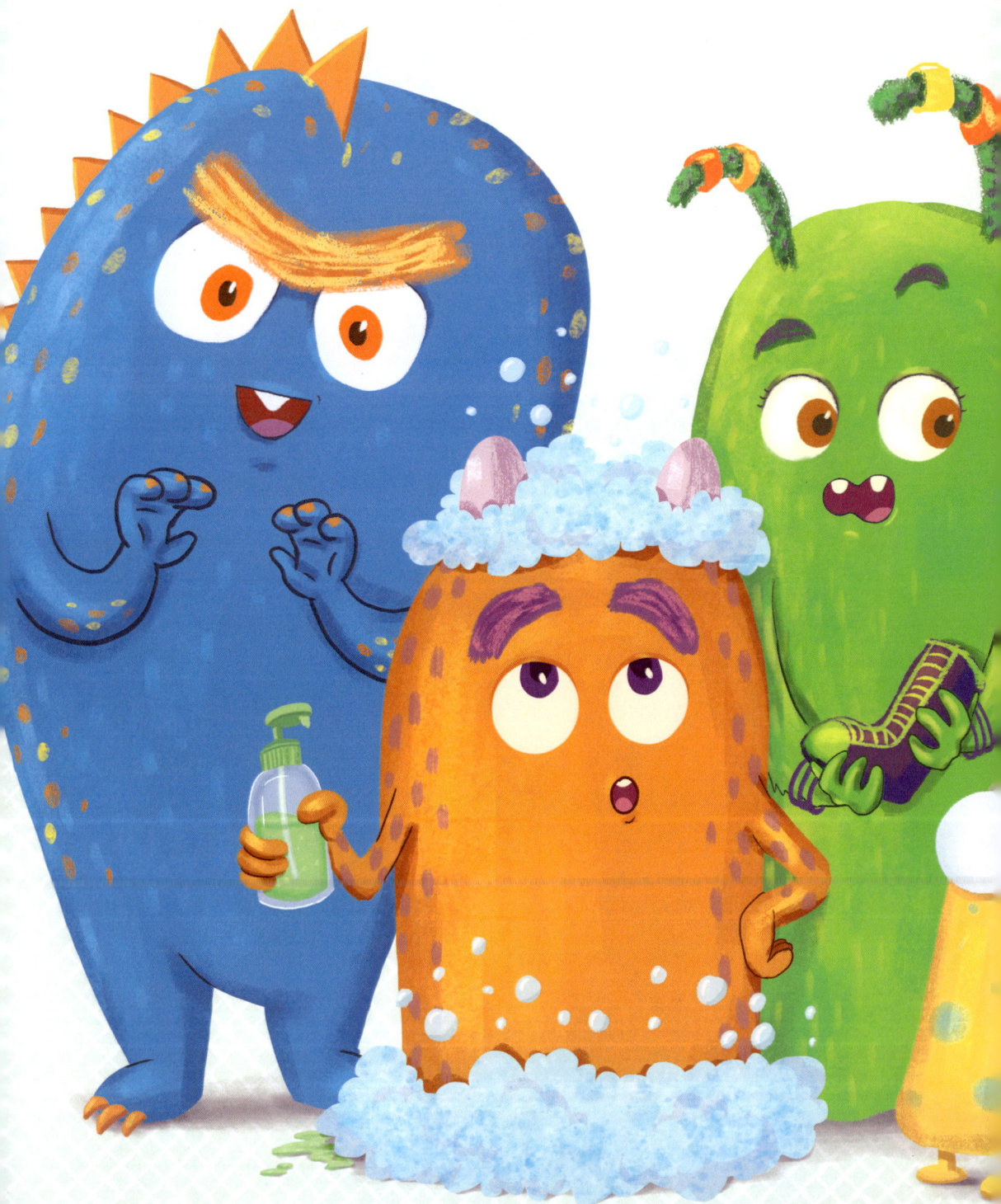

But Worry Monster makes our scary thoughts
bigger than they are,
And takes our normal thoughts
and makes them totally bizarre.

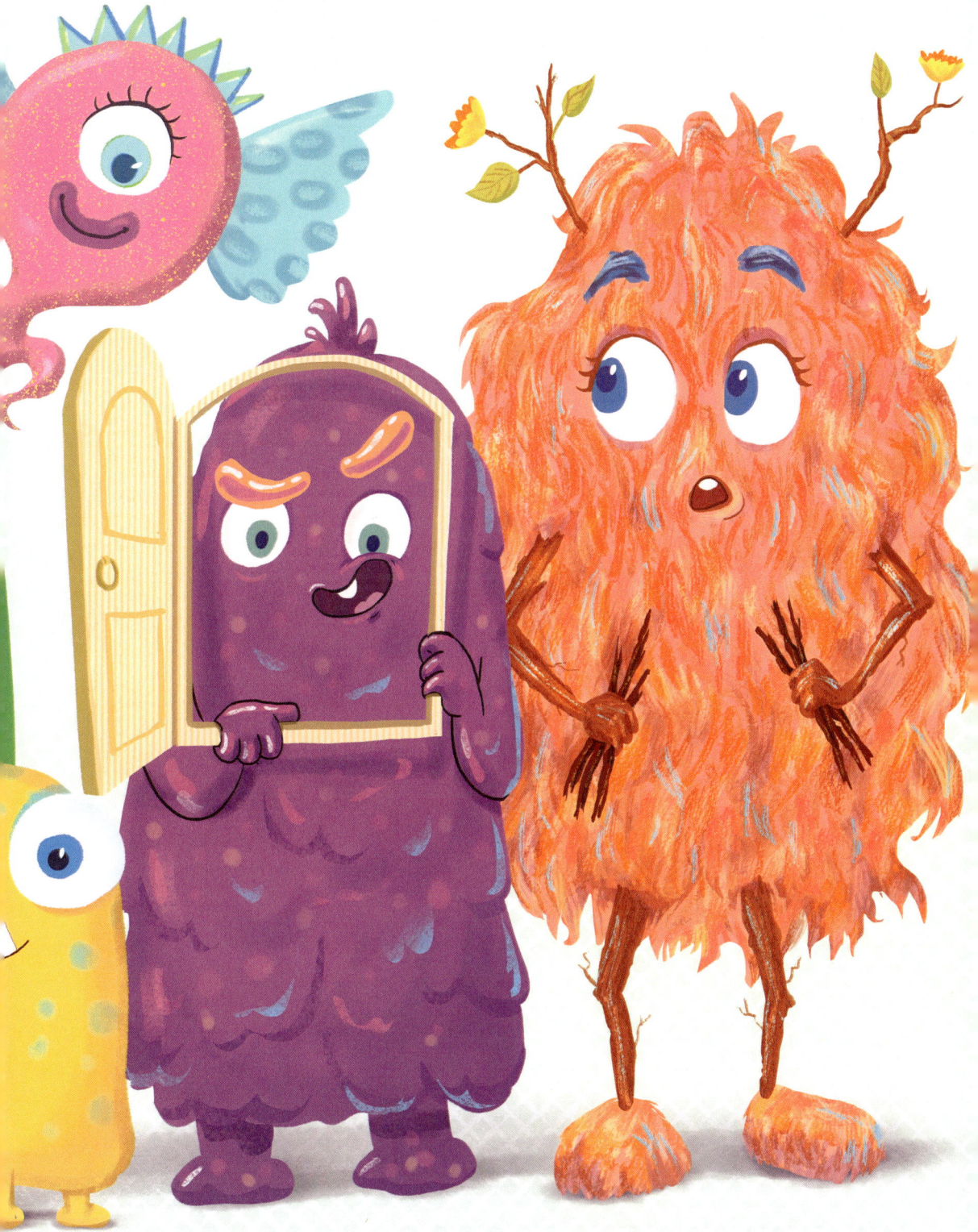

Zara was a girl who was curious and sweet,
She was born with very special feet.

When her Worry Monster talked,
it made her feel so wrong.
Her Worry Monster tried to tell her
she was never strong.

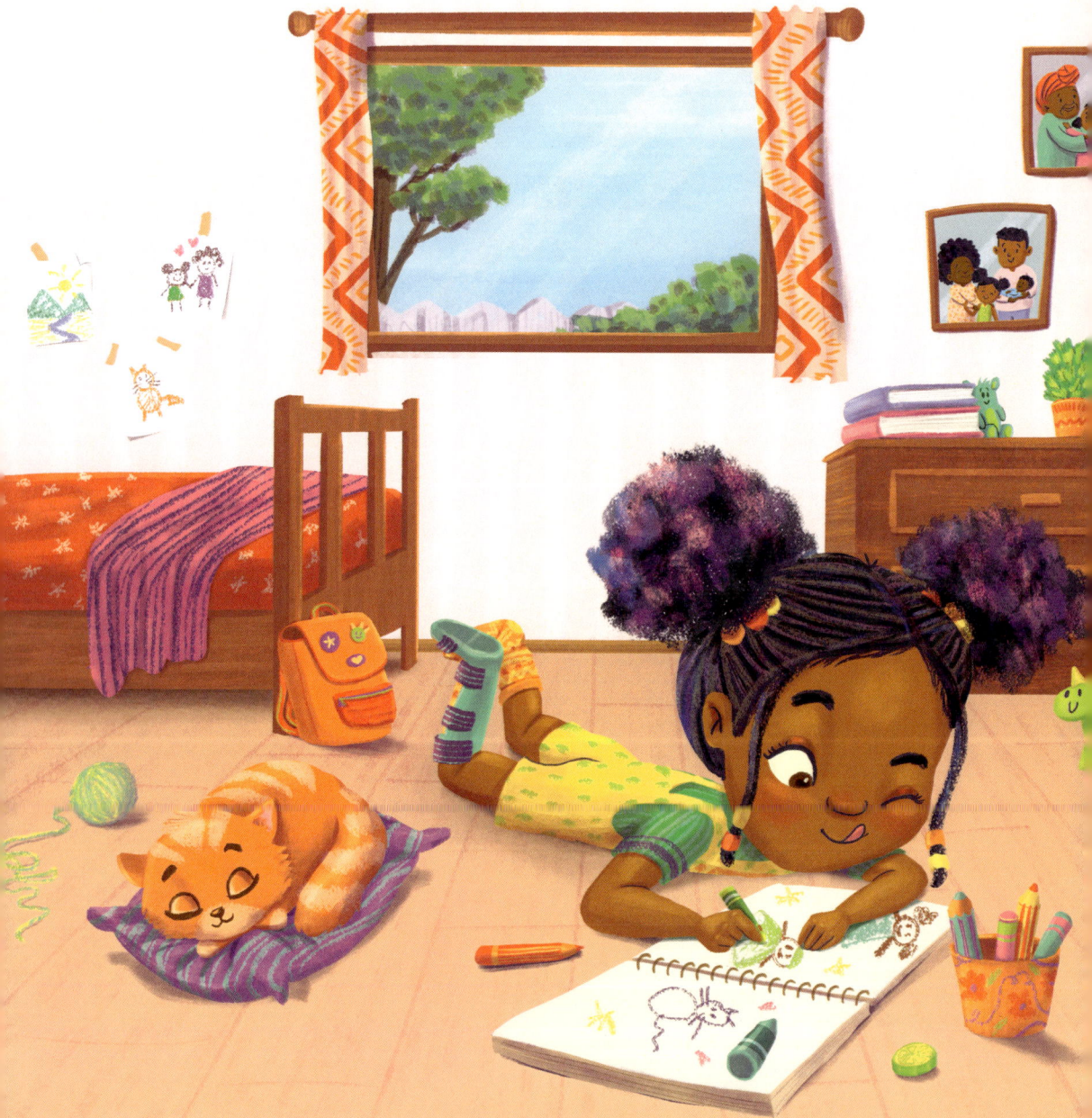

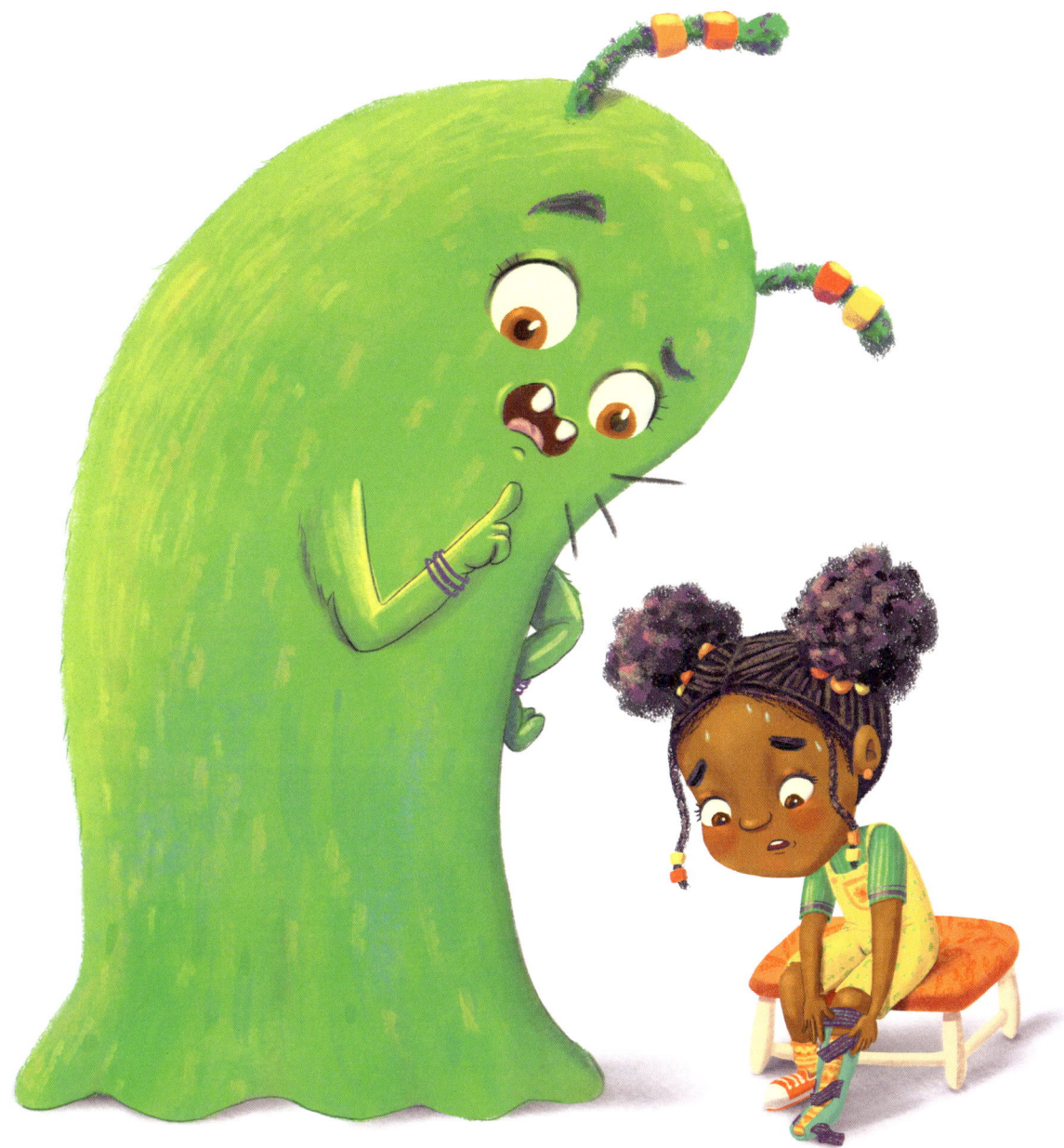

One, Two, Buckle Your Shoe,
This is the Worry Monster Talking to You.

If you don't listen
and do what I say,
You'll be thinking this thought
all through the day!

But Zara was wise and stood up tall,
She did not have to listen to the monster at all.

"What ever you say is NOT what I'll do!
Worry Monster, I don't listen to you!"

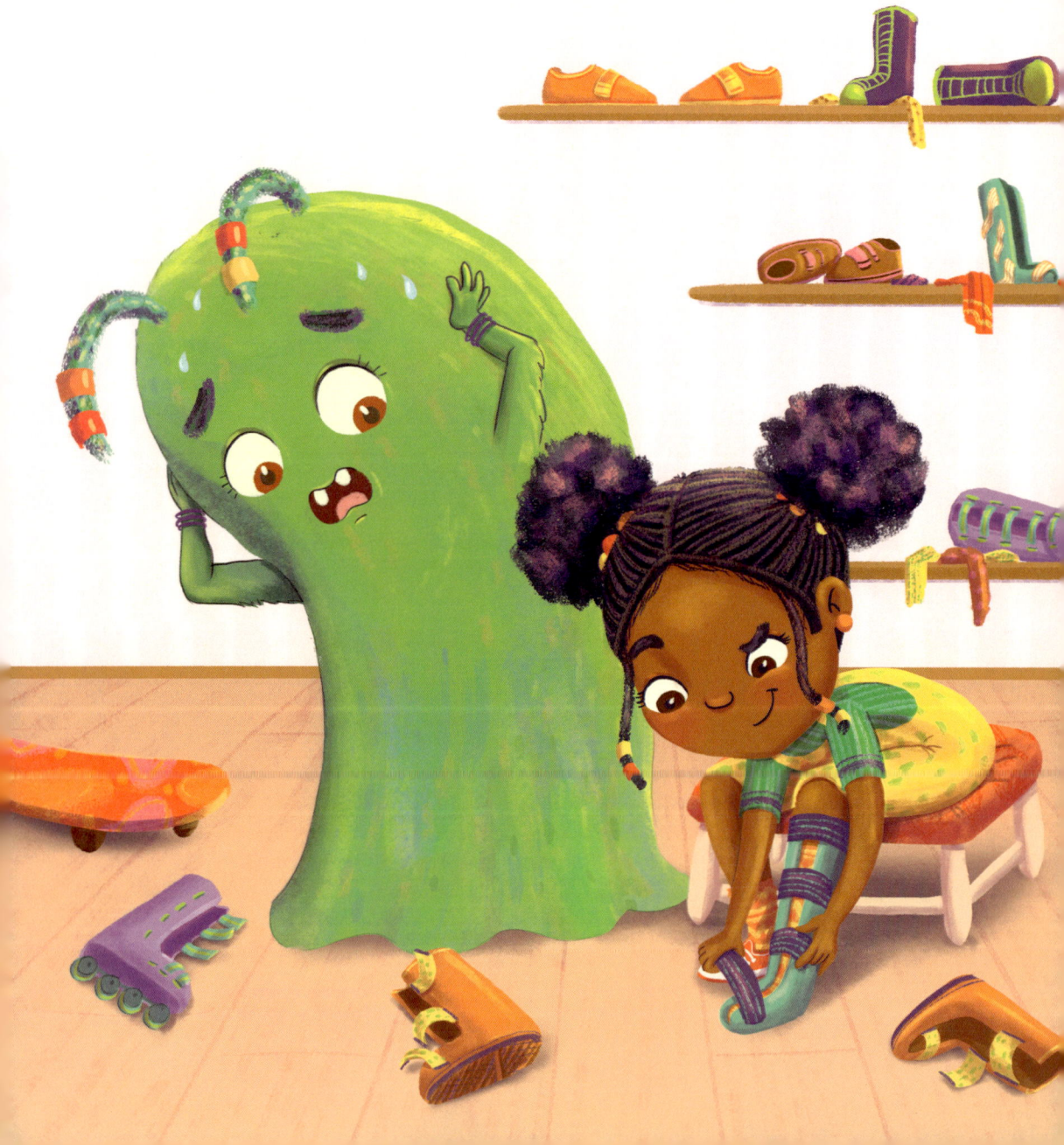

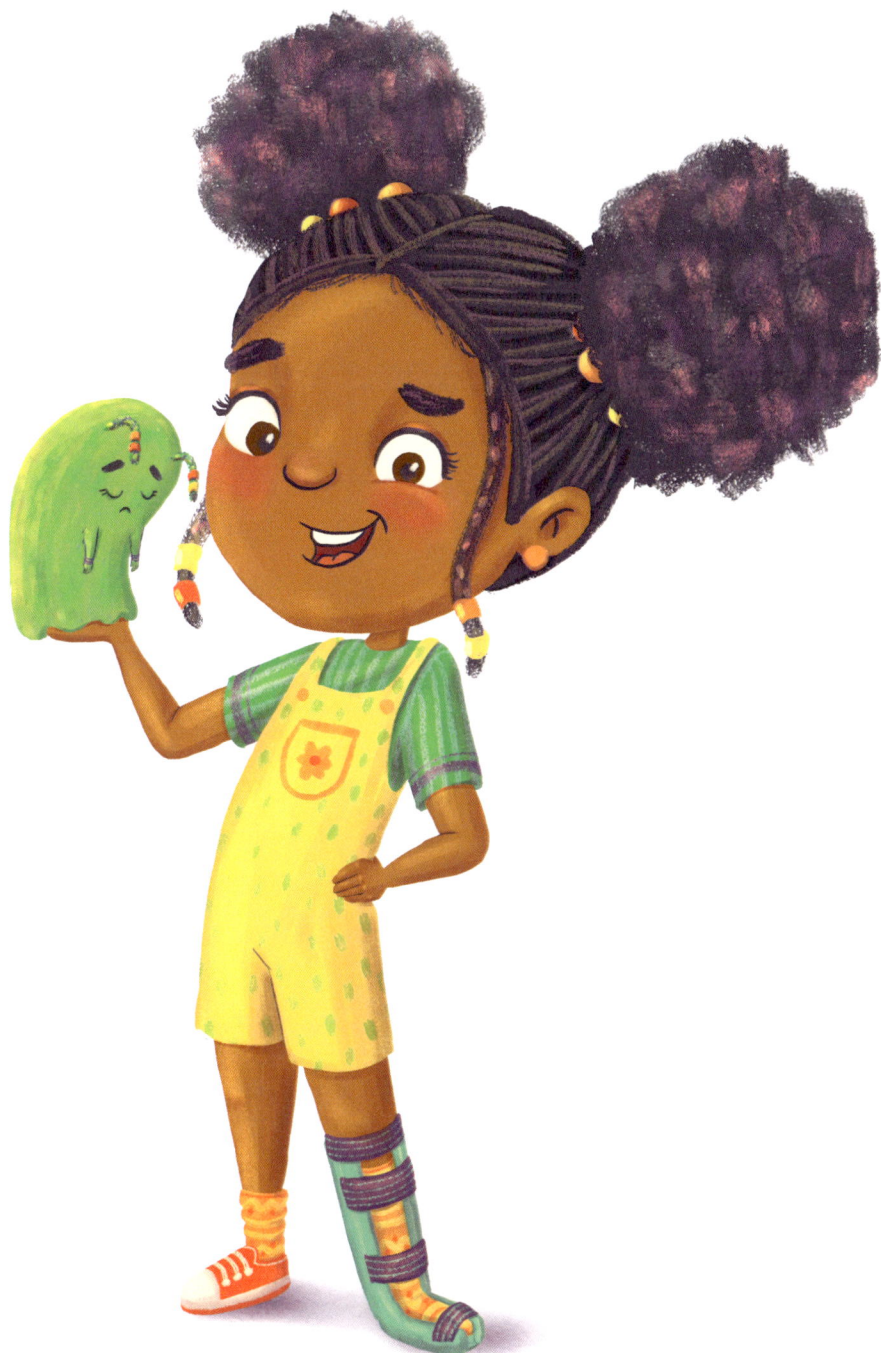

Talking back made
the Worry Monster shake,
Zara knew winning
was a piece of cake.

Finn was a boy who was kind and smart,
And his superpower was his amazing heart.

But when his Worry Monster came to play,
Finn was not the same all day.

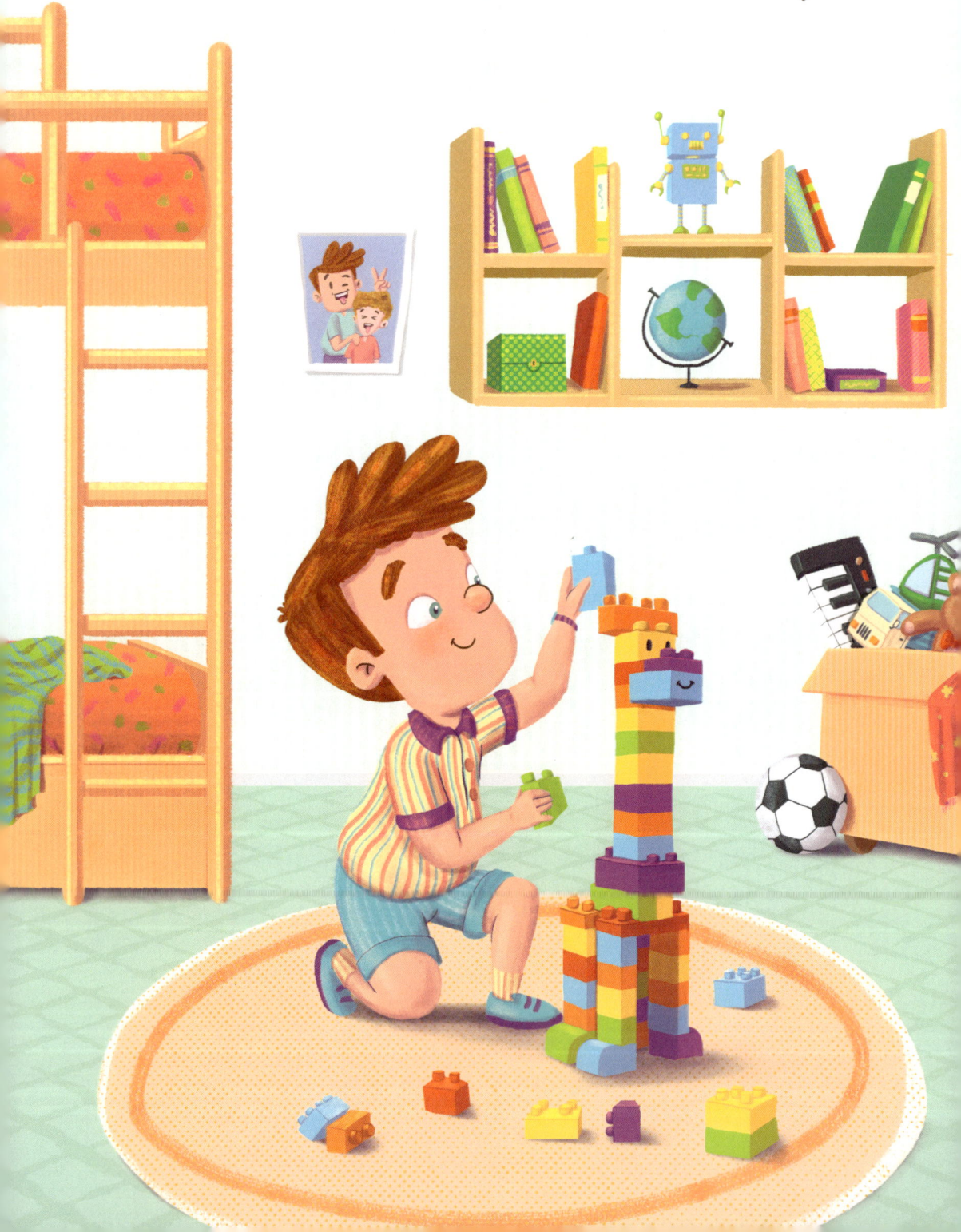

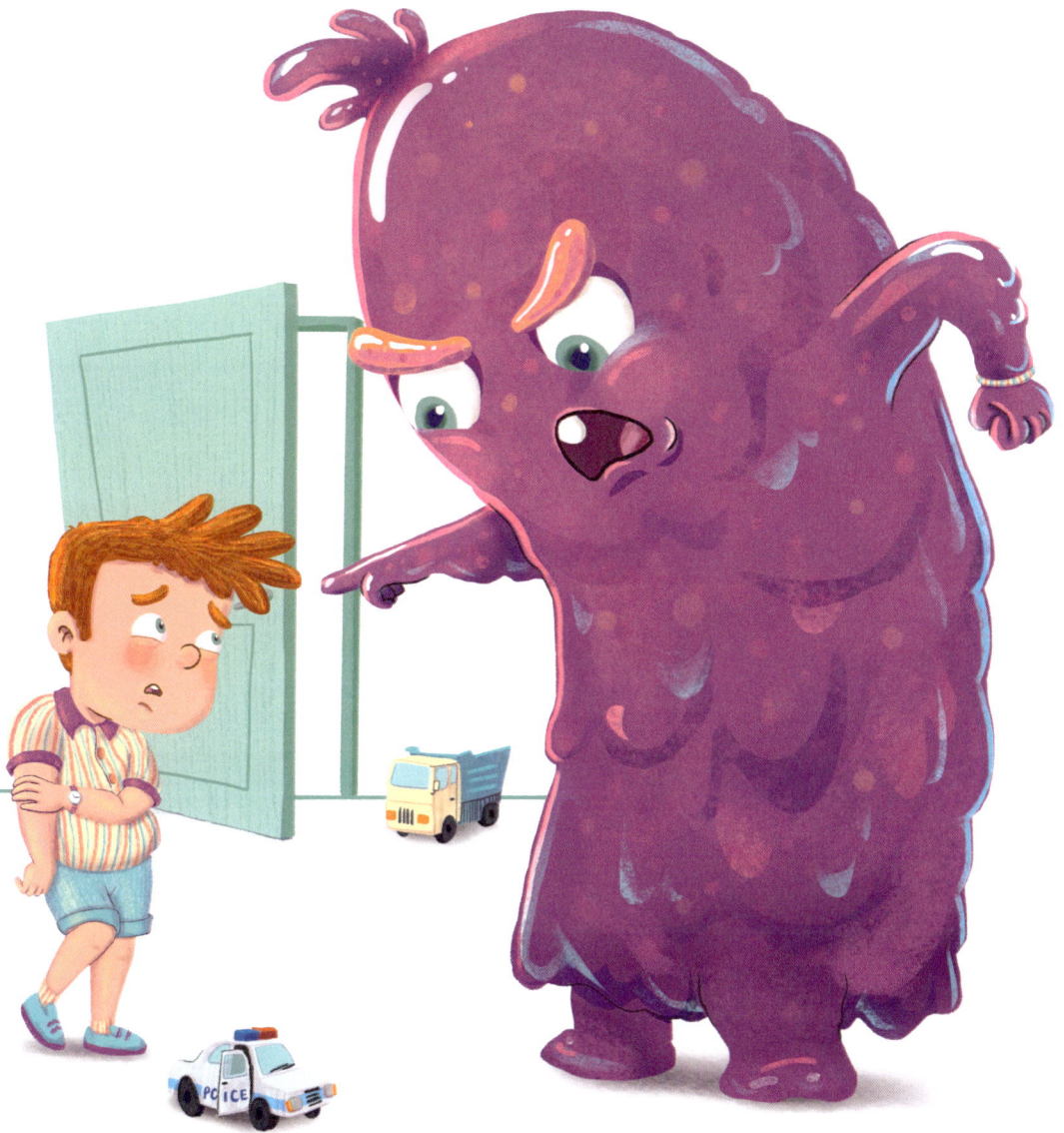

Three, Four,
Shut the Door
Open them, shut them,
that's what they're for.

If you don't do as I say -
That door will bother you all day!

Finn was nervous and scared to play,
But then he remembered what his mom would say.

"I'll open and leave it or close it all wrong.
Worry Monster you're not really all that strong!"

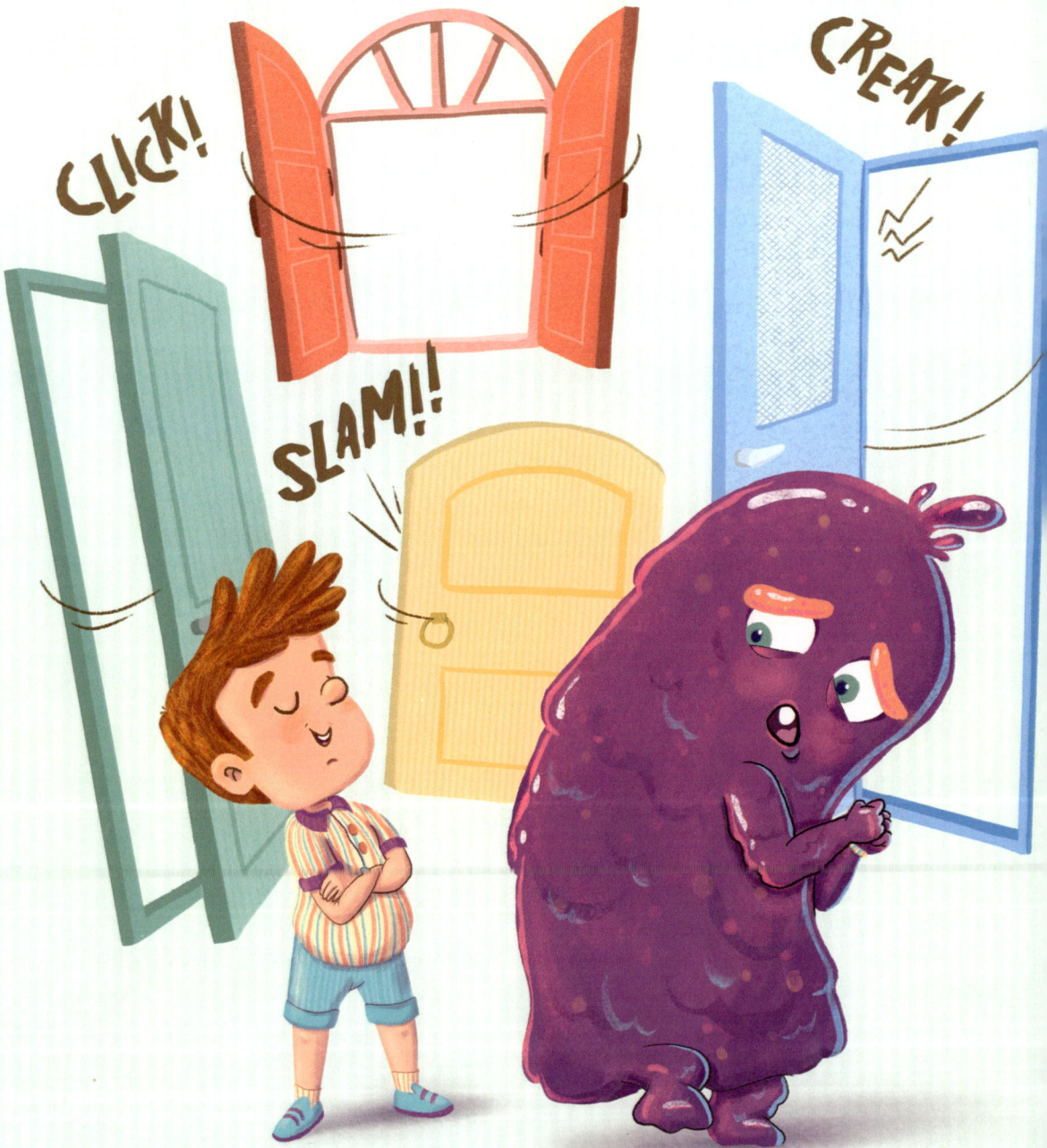

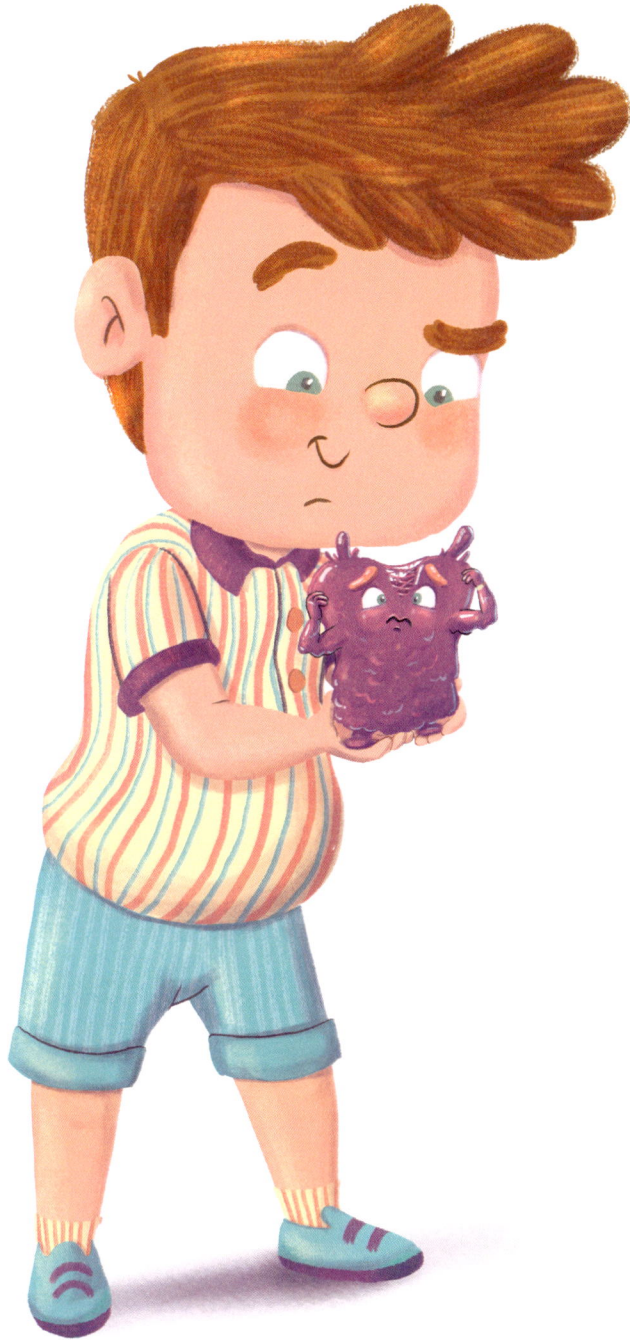

Worry Monster didn't like that one bit,
Doing things different made him want to split.

Sophia was clever and quick, it's true,
Her brain loved numbers and math problems too.

But her Worry Monster loved 3, 7, and 9,
And made Sophia feel like nothing was fine.

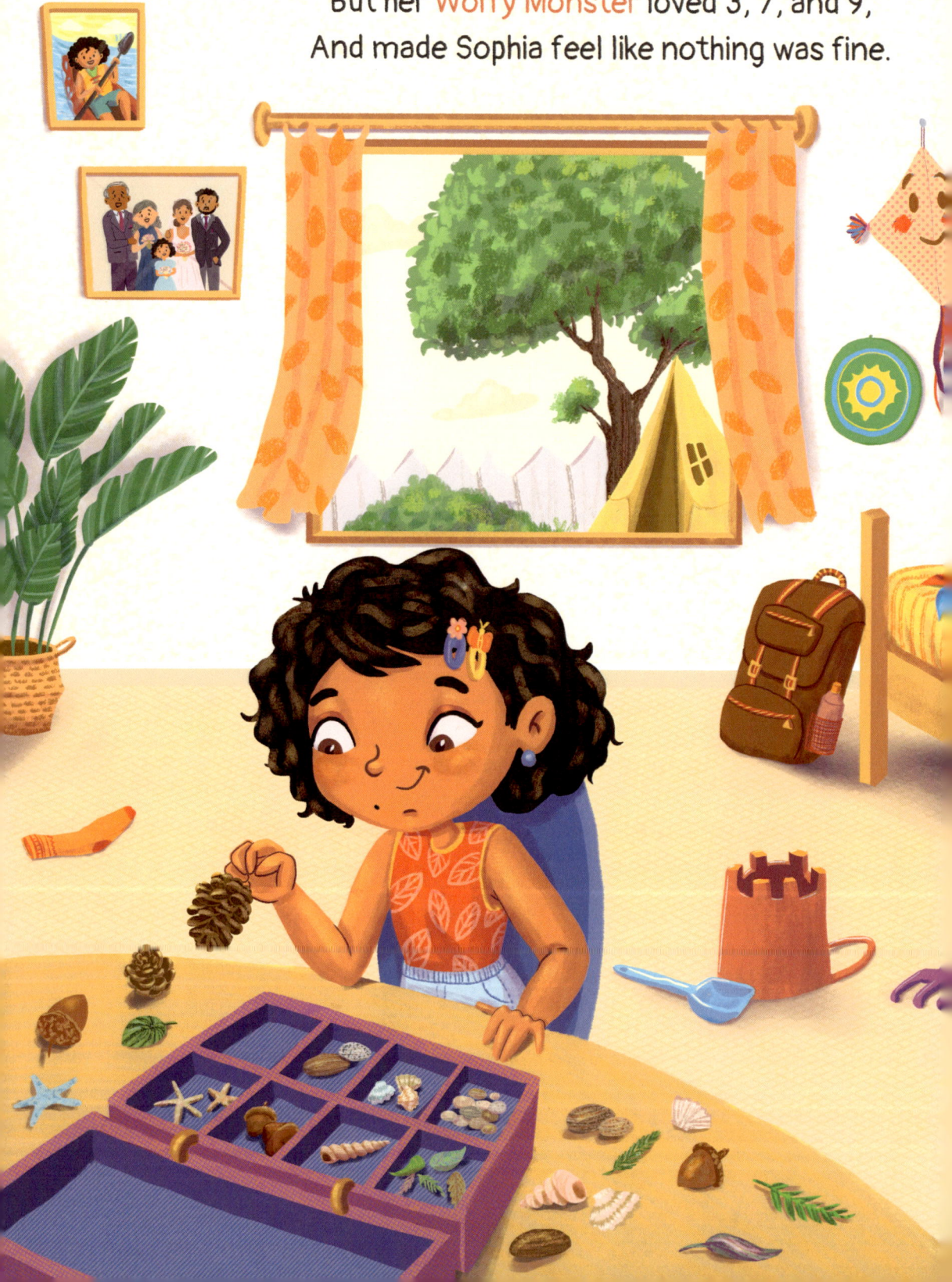

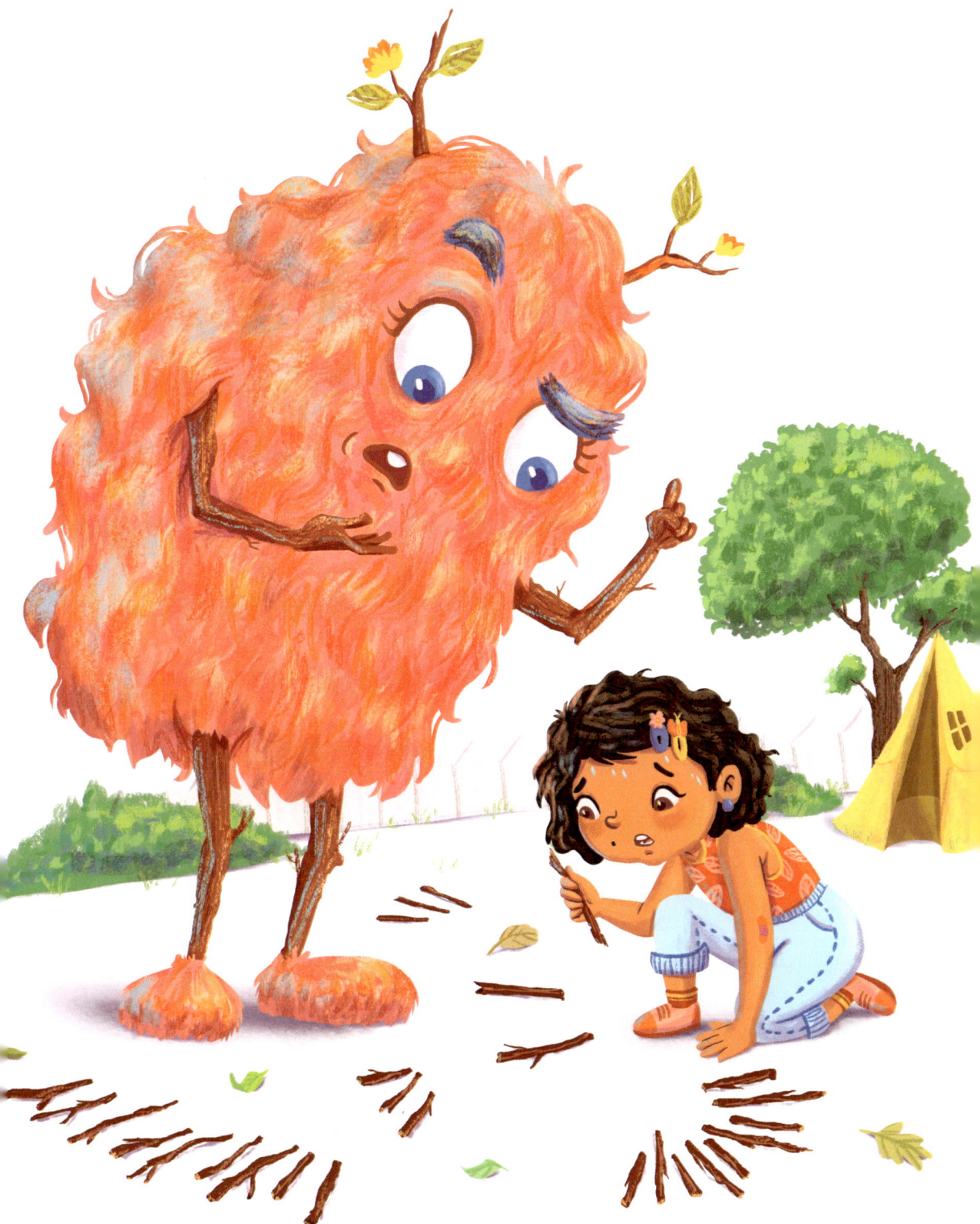

Five, Six, Pick up Sticks,
Sort them, count them, fall for my tricks.
If you don't listen, you'll know what I'll do,
I'll keep mixing up numbers and worrying you!

Sophia was scared, shaky, and sour,
But she remembered her secret superpower.

"Worry Monster, I know that I'm smarter than you,
I just have to do what you CAN'T do!"

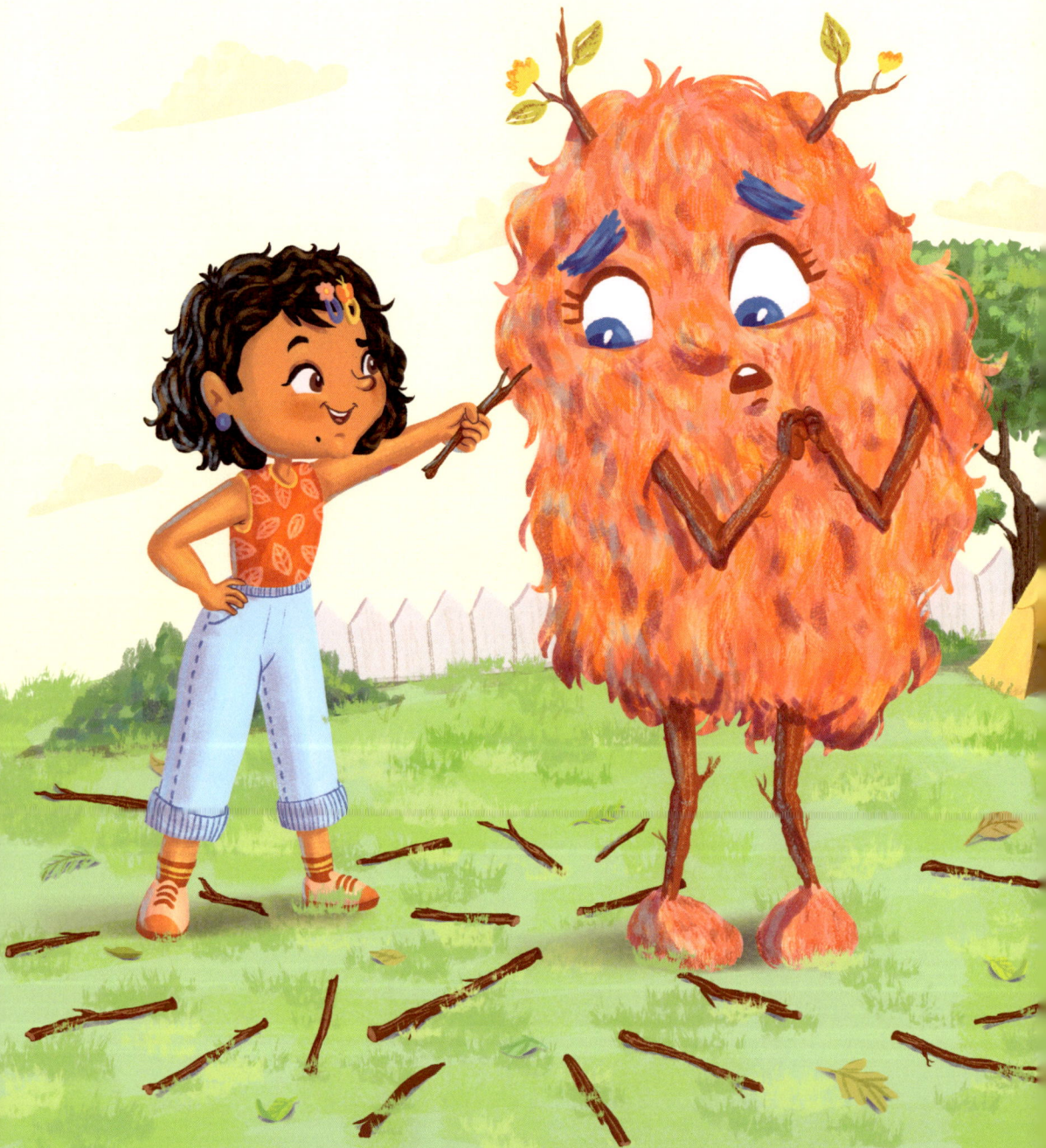

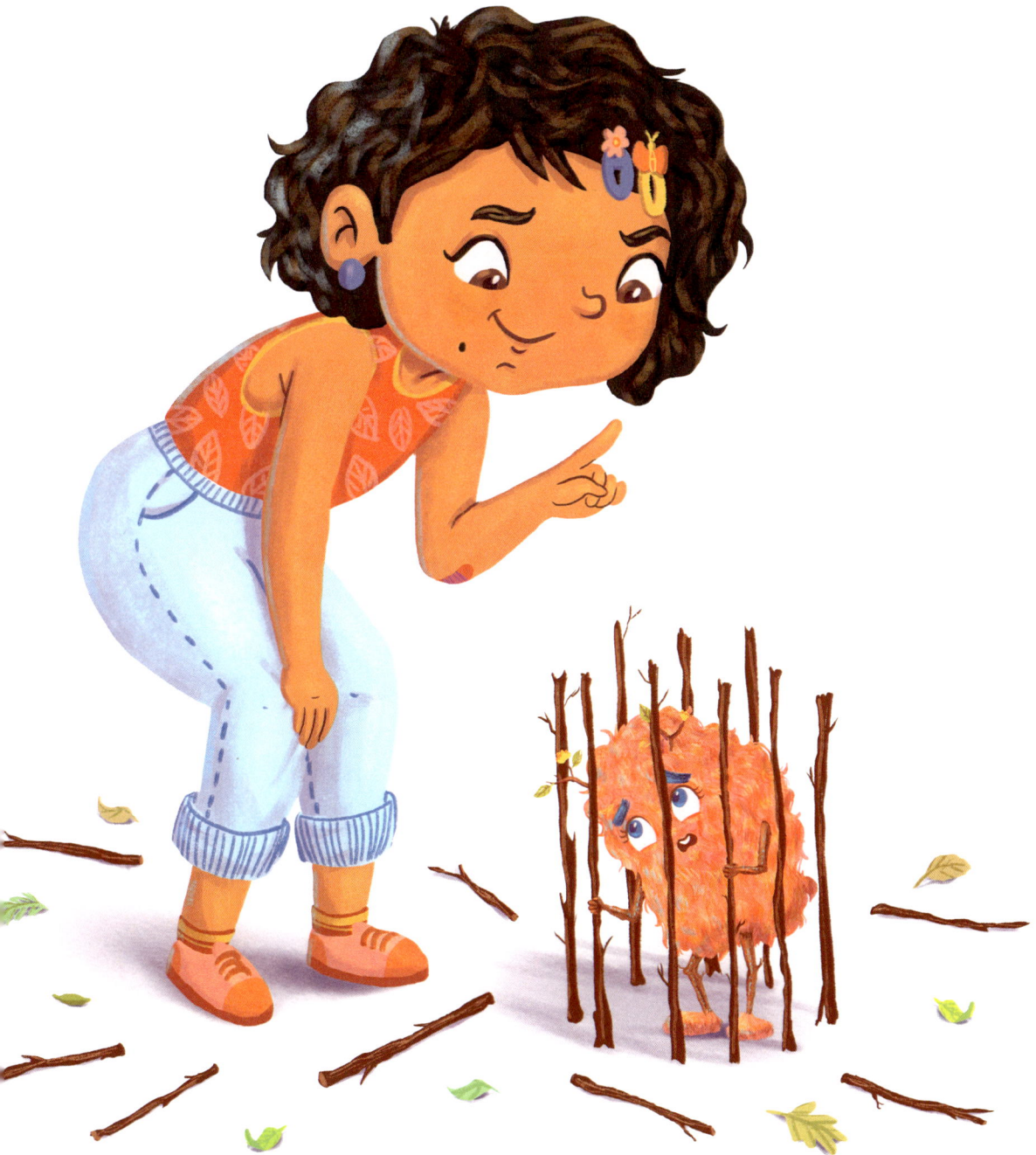

She watched Worry Monster squirm and wriggle,
Beating him made Sophia giggle.

Shah was a boy who was daring and cool,
He loved cars and his friends at school.

But Worry Monster had him beat,
He told Shah to be perfectly neat.

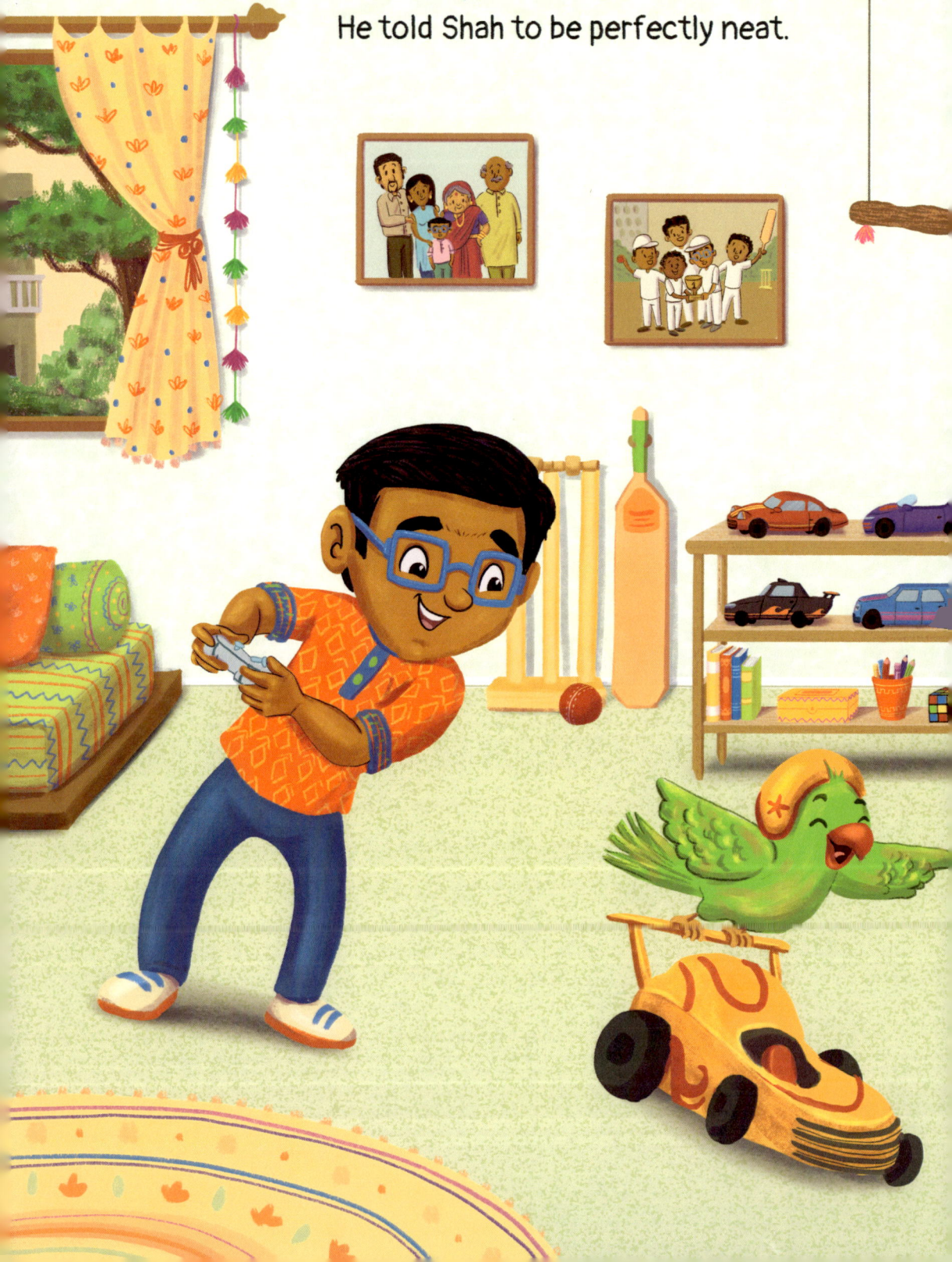

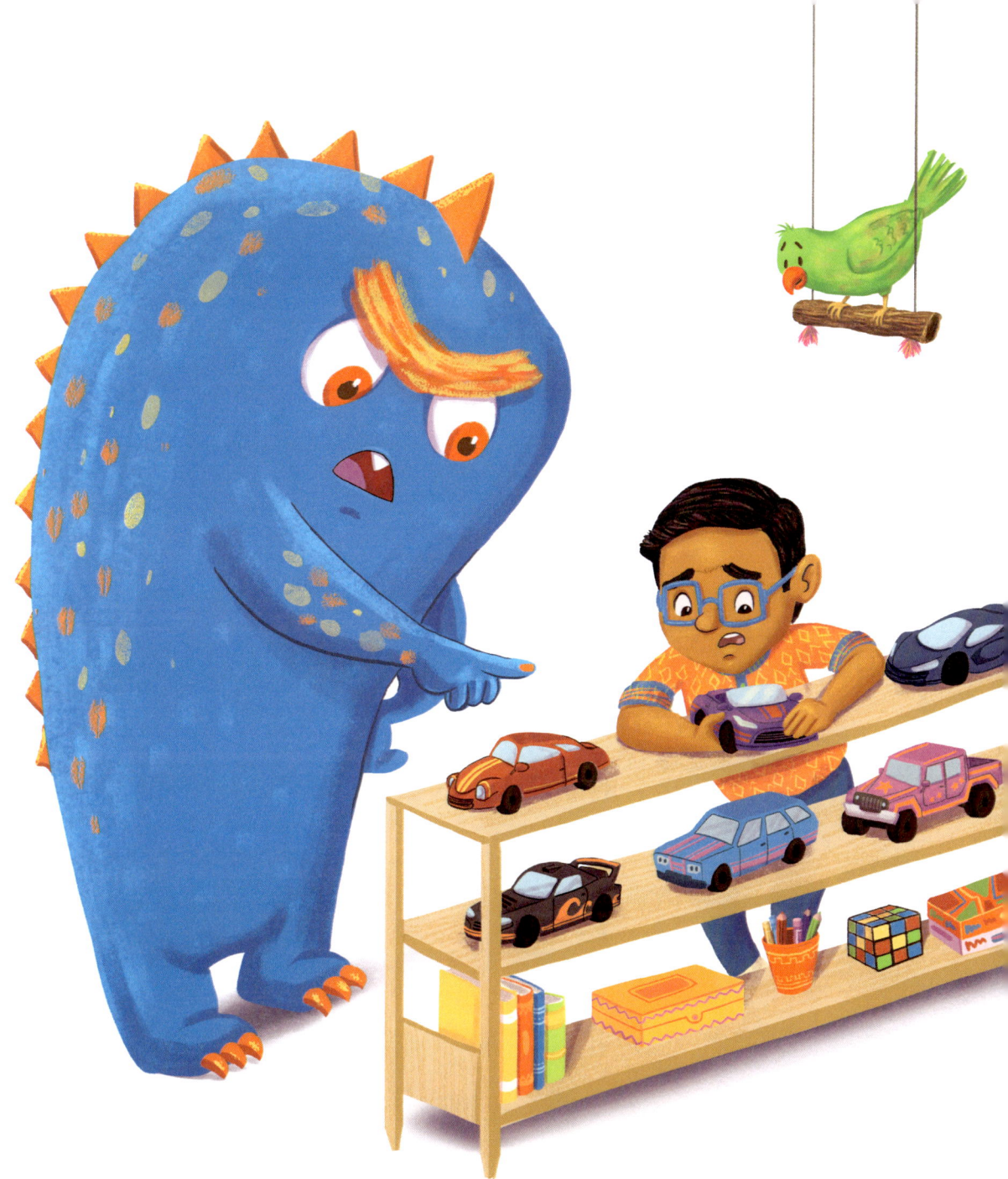

Seven, Eight, Lay Them Straight,
Keep them perfect and don't be late.

If you can't fix them up just right,
I'll stay in your thoughts throughout the night!

Worried thoughts swirled around in his head,
But Shah wanted to feel safe in his bed.

"Worry Monster, you lie and take things too far,
I know I am stronger than you are!"

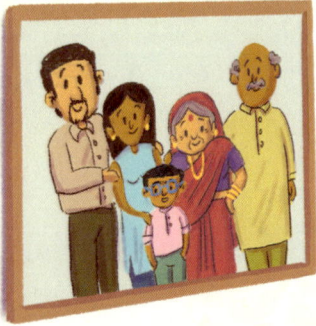

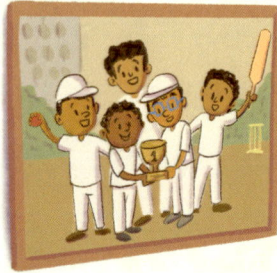

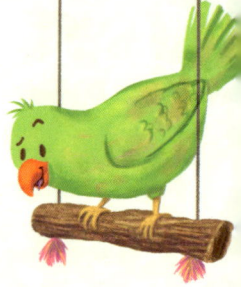

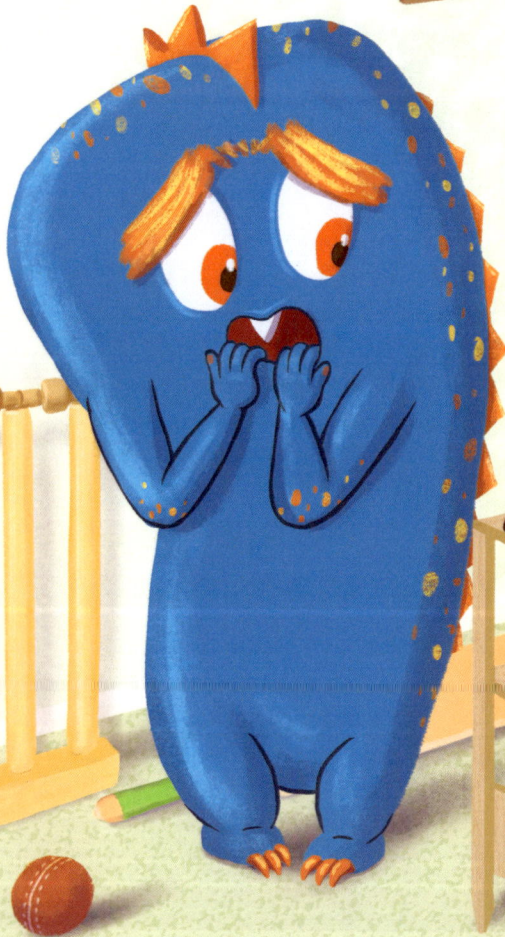

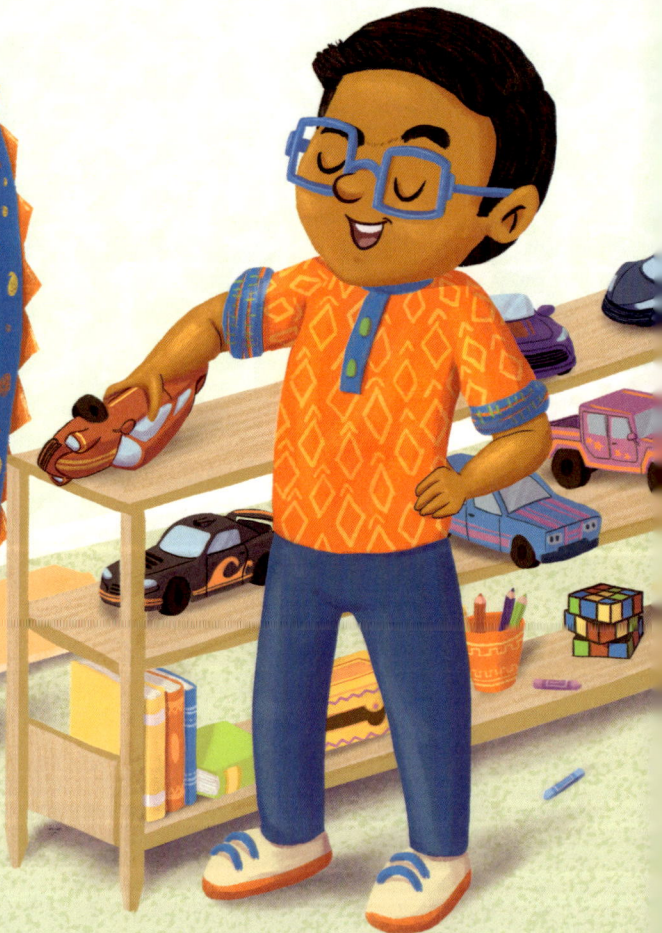

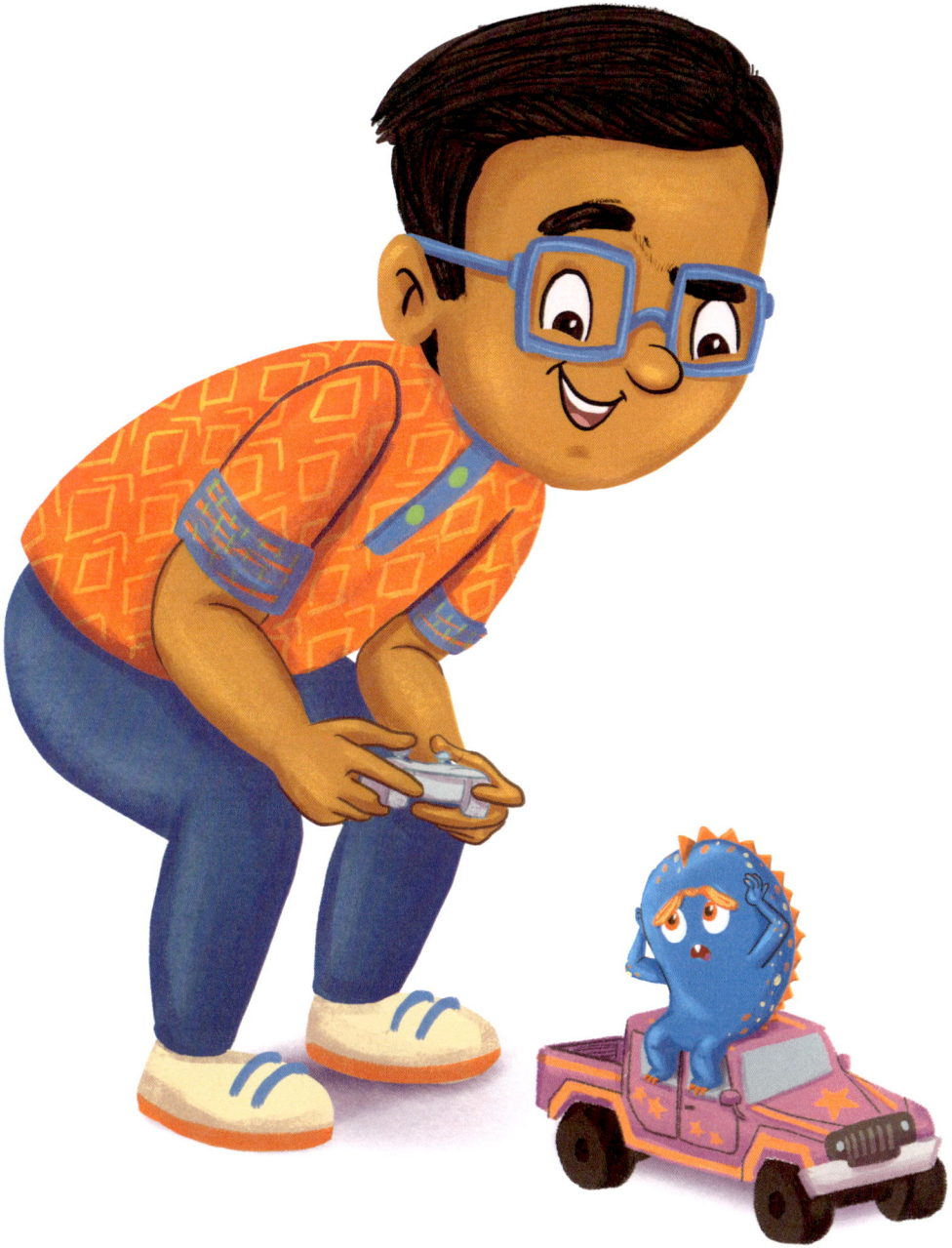

Worry Monster was bested - he was done,
Shah knew that the battle was won.

Jayden was creative and fun,
He always had a smile for everyone.

But Worry Monster told him he was not clean,
Worry Monster said things that were really mean.

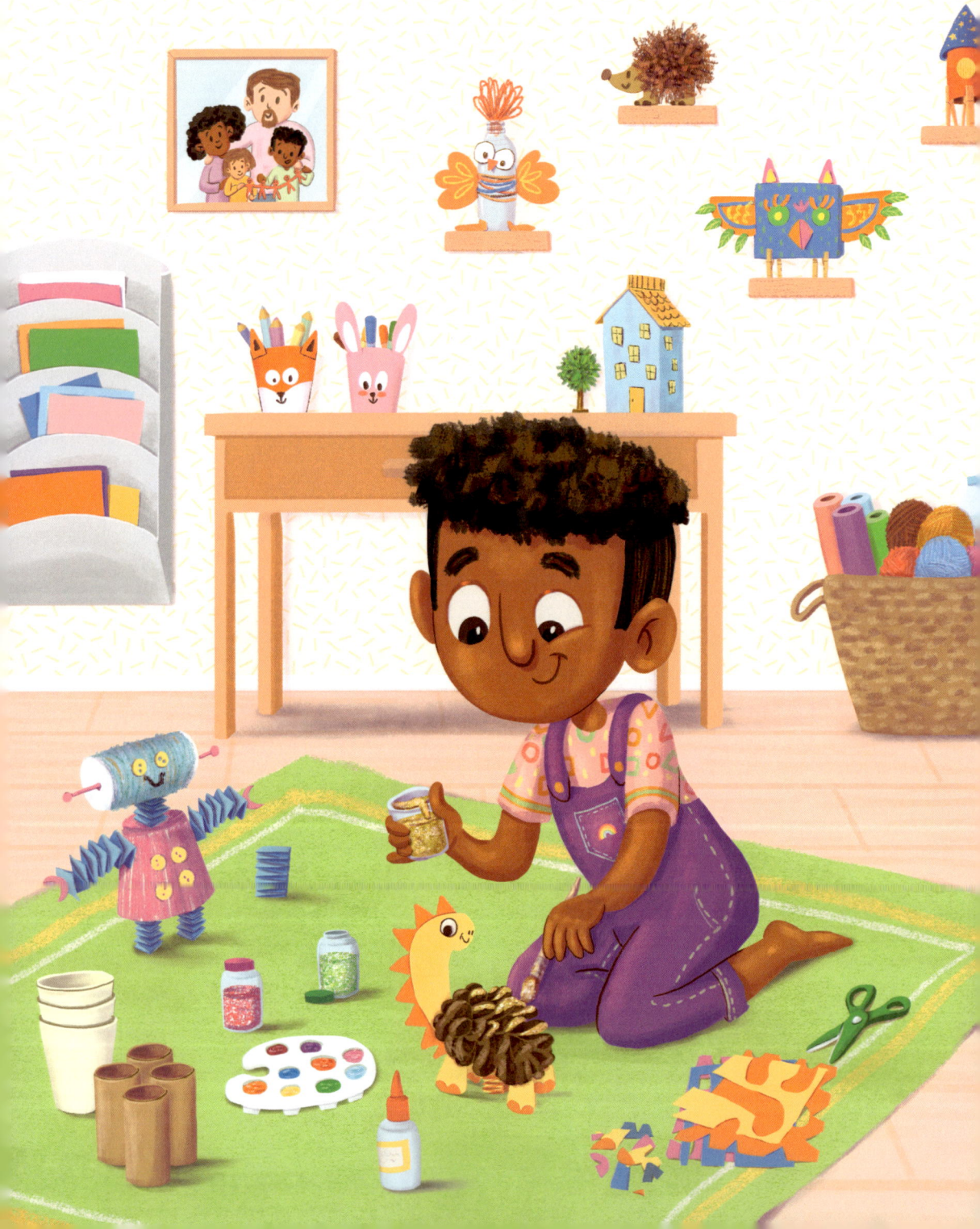

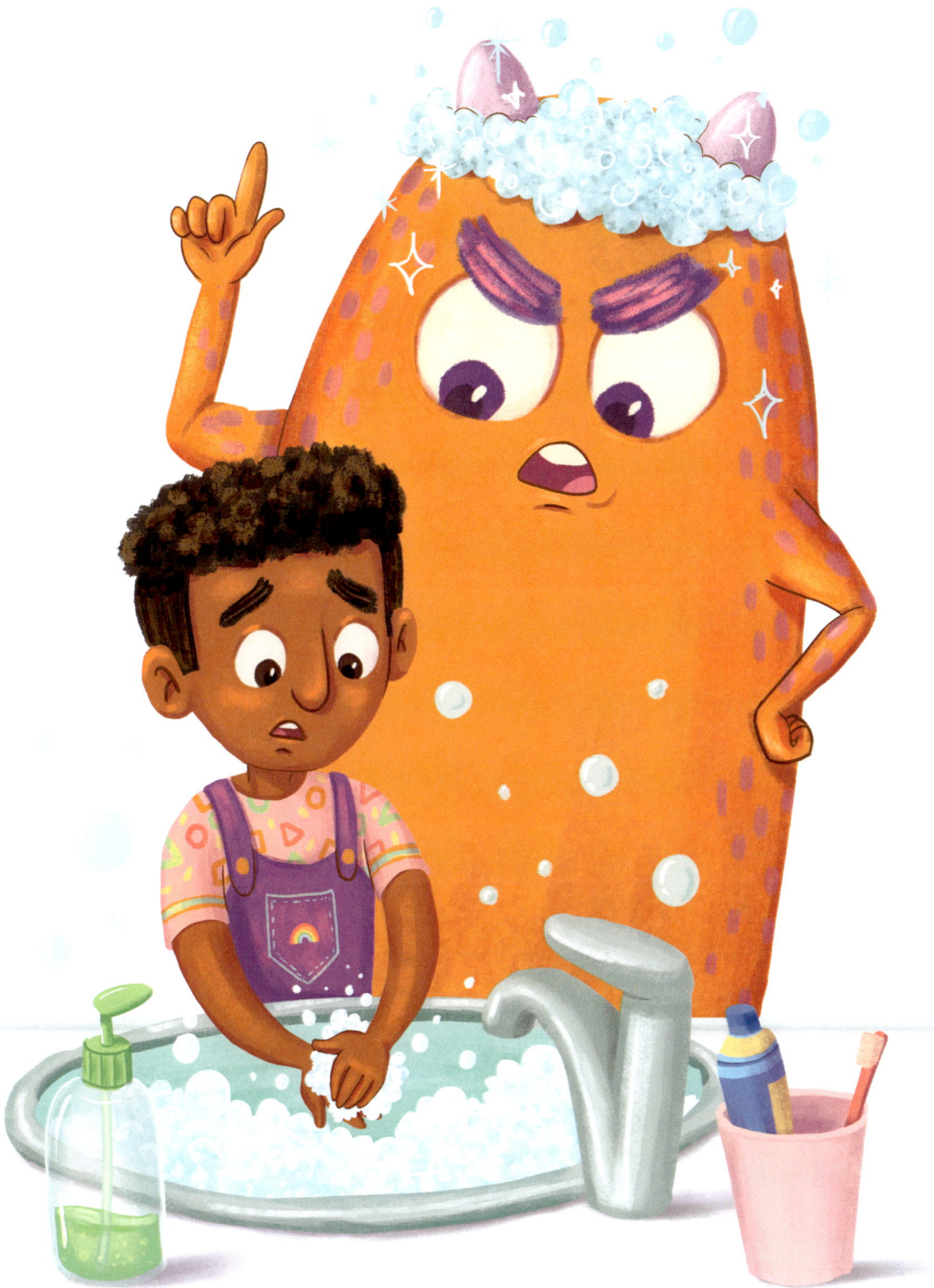

Nine, Ten, Do it Again!
Again and Again until I say when!
If you don't listen to all that I do,
These worried thoughts will keep coming to you!

Worry Monster's taunts filled Jayden with dread,
Until his father's words rang in his head.

"My hands may be dirty and have germs too,
But that doesn't mean I should listen to you!"

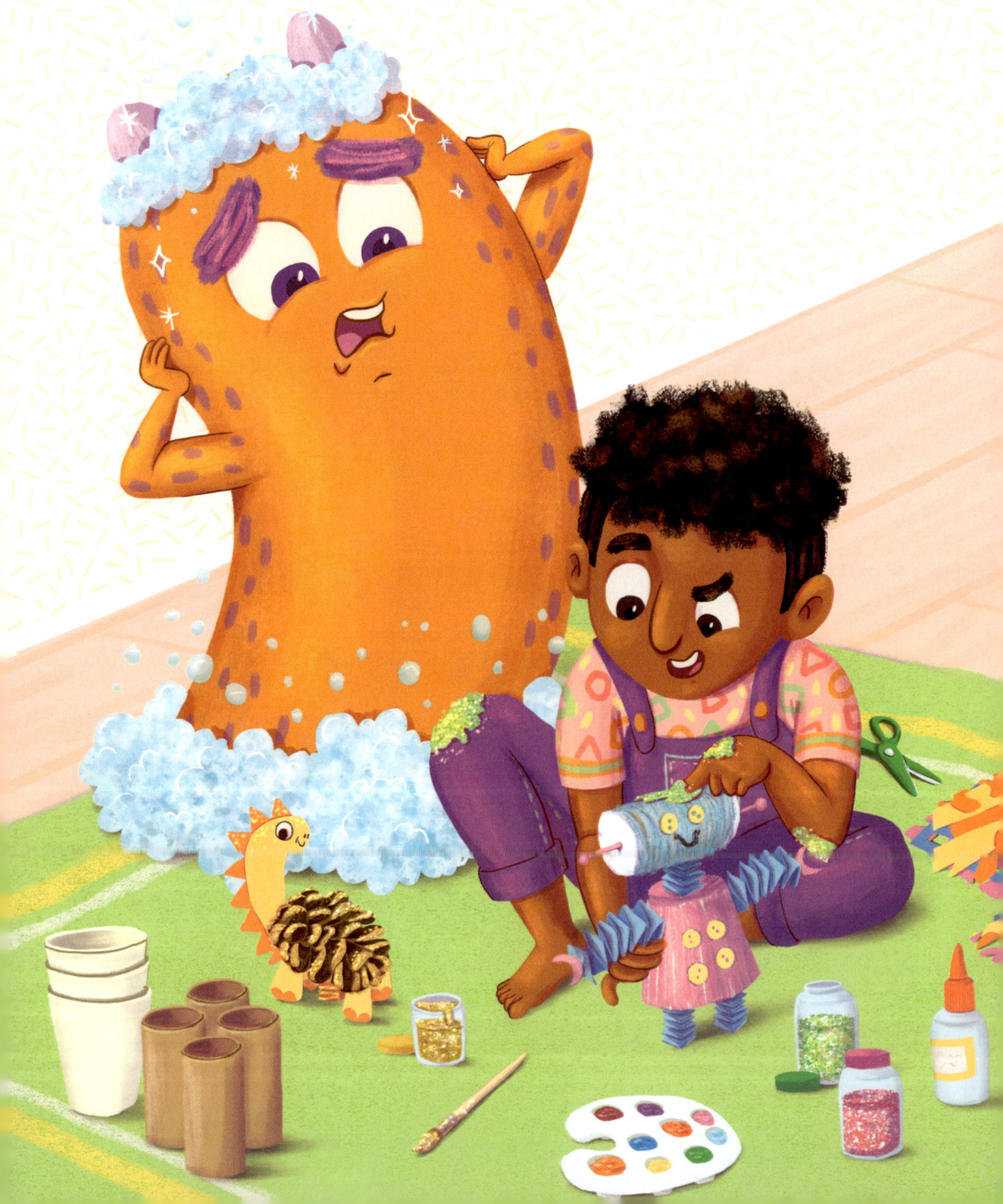

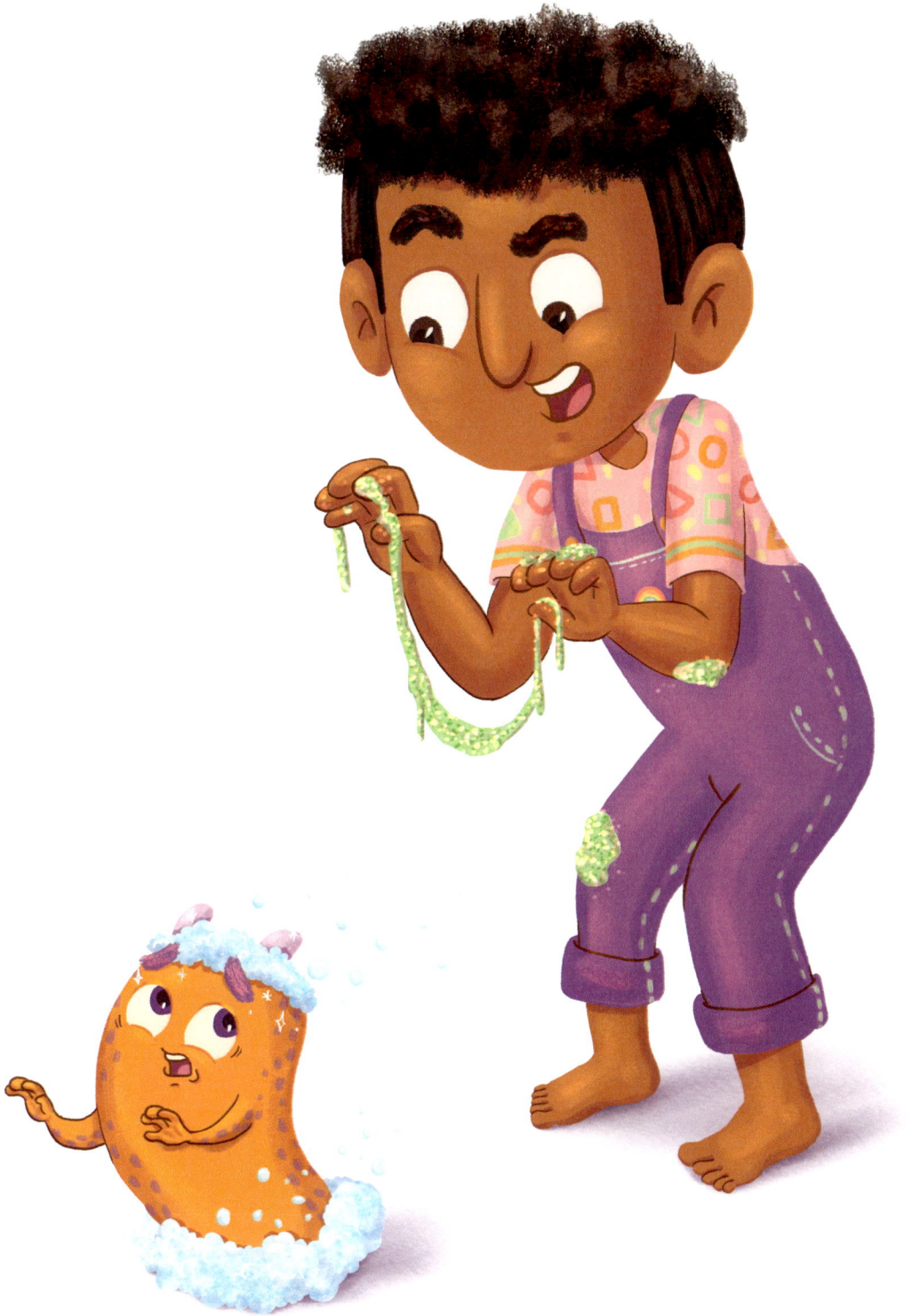

Worry Monster didn't like that at all!
He was shrinking, he had become so small!

So when your Worry Monster is acting out,
Or yelling, or screaming, or making you doubt,
You don't have to listen to whatever it said,
You can do something different instead.

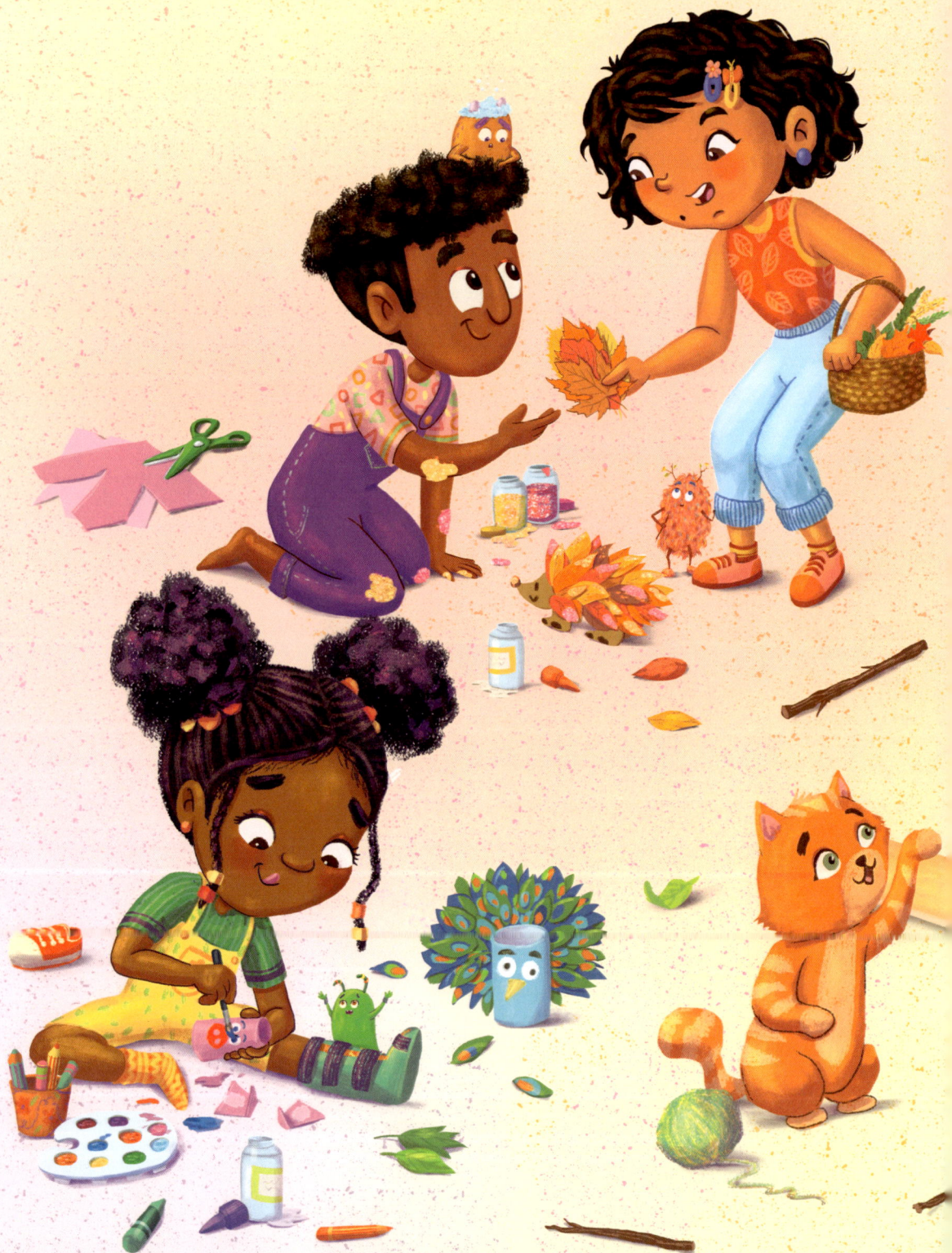

Challenge them, push them, sing a silly song,
Make your Worry Monster feel all wrong.
Whatever you try and whatever you do,
Make your Worry Monster listen to YOU!

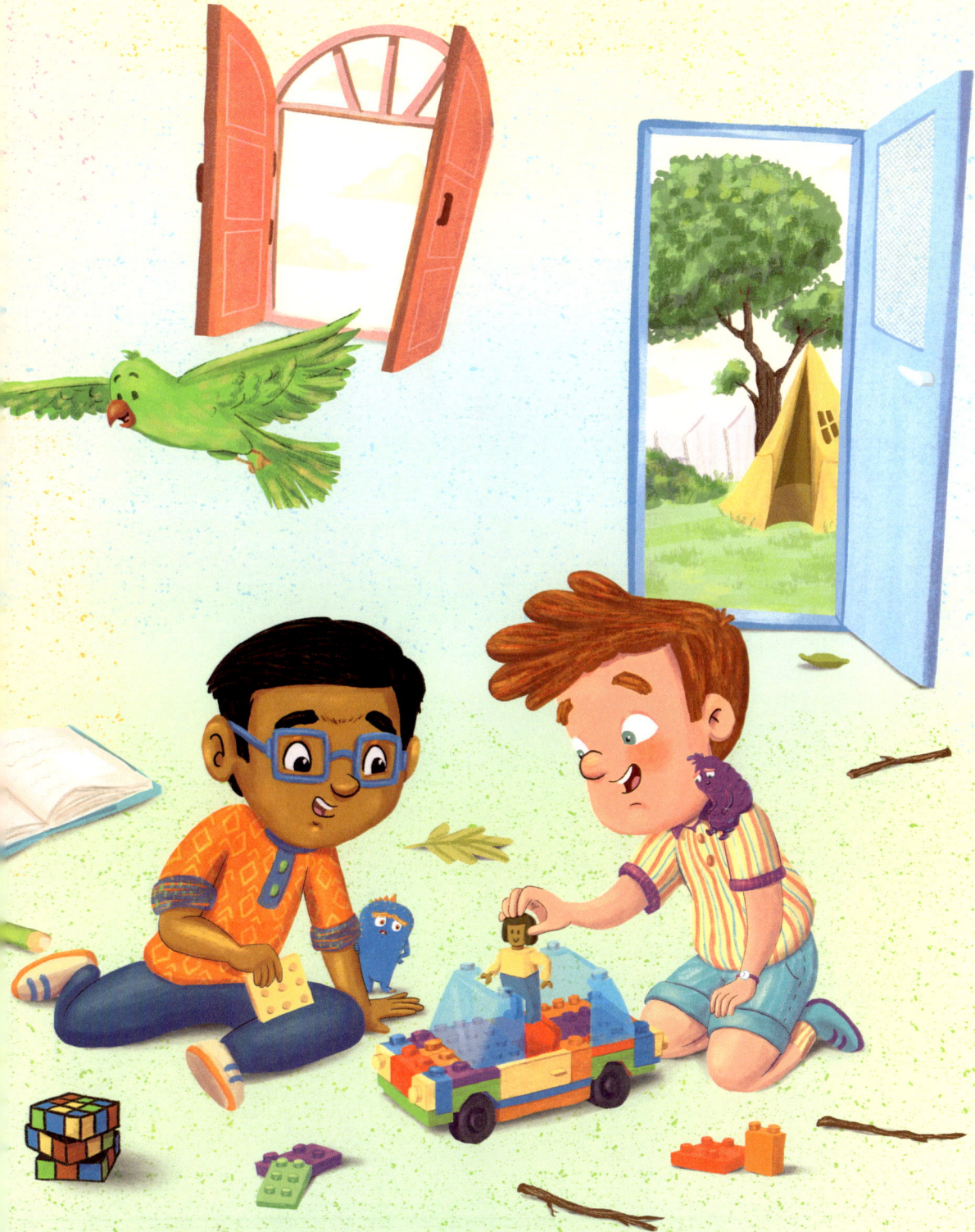

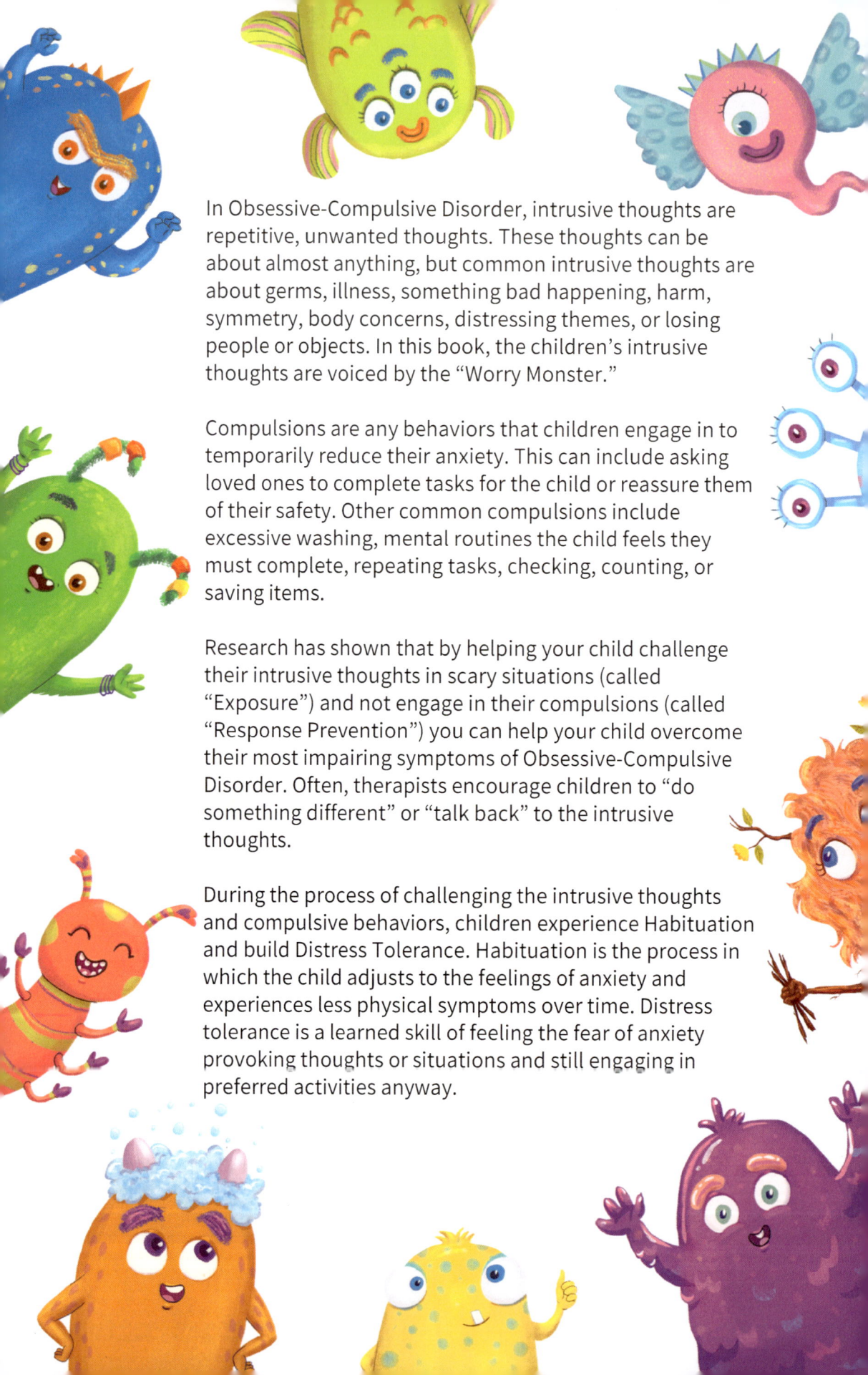

In Obsessive-Compulsive Disorder, intrusive thoughts are repetitive, unwanted thoughts. These thoughts can be about almost anything, but common intrusive thoughts are about germs, illness, something bad happening, harm, symmetry, body concerns, distressing themes, or losing people or objects. In this book, the children's intrusive thoughts are voiced by the "Worry Monster."

Compulsions are any behaviors that children engage in to temporarily reduce their anxiety. This can include asking loved ones to complete tasks for the child or reassure them of their safety. Other common compulsions include excessive washing, mental routines the child feels they must complete, repeating tasks, checking, counting, or saving items.

Research has shown that by helping your child challenge their intrusive thoughts in scary situations (called "Exposure") and not engage in their compulsions (called "Response Prevention") you can help your child overcome their most impairing symptoms of Obsessive-Compulsive Disorder. Often, therapists encourage children to "do something different" or "talk back" to the intrusive thoughts.

During the process of challenging the intrusive thoughts and compulsive behaviors, children experience Habituation and build Distress Tolerance. Habituation is the process in which the child adjusts to the feelings of anxiety and experiences less physical symptoms over time. Distress tolerance is a learned skill of feeling the fear of anxiety provoking thoughts or situations and still engaging in preferred activities anyway.

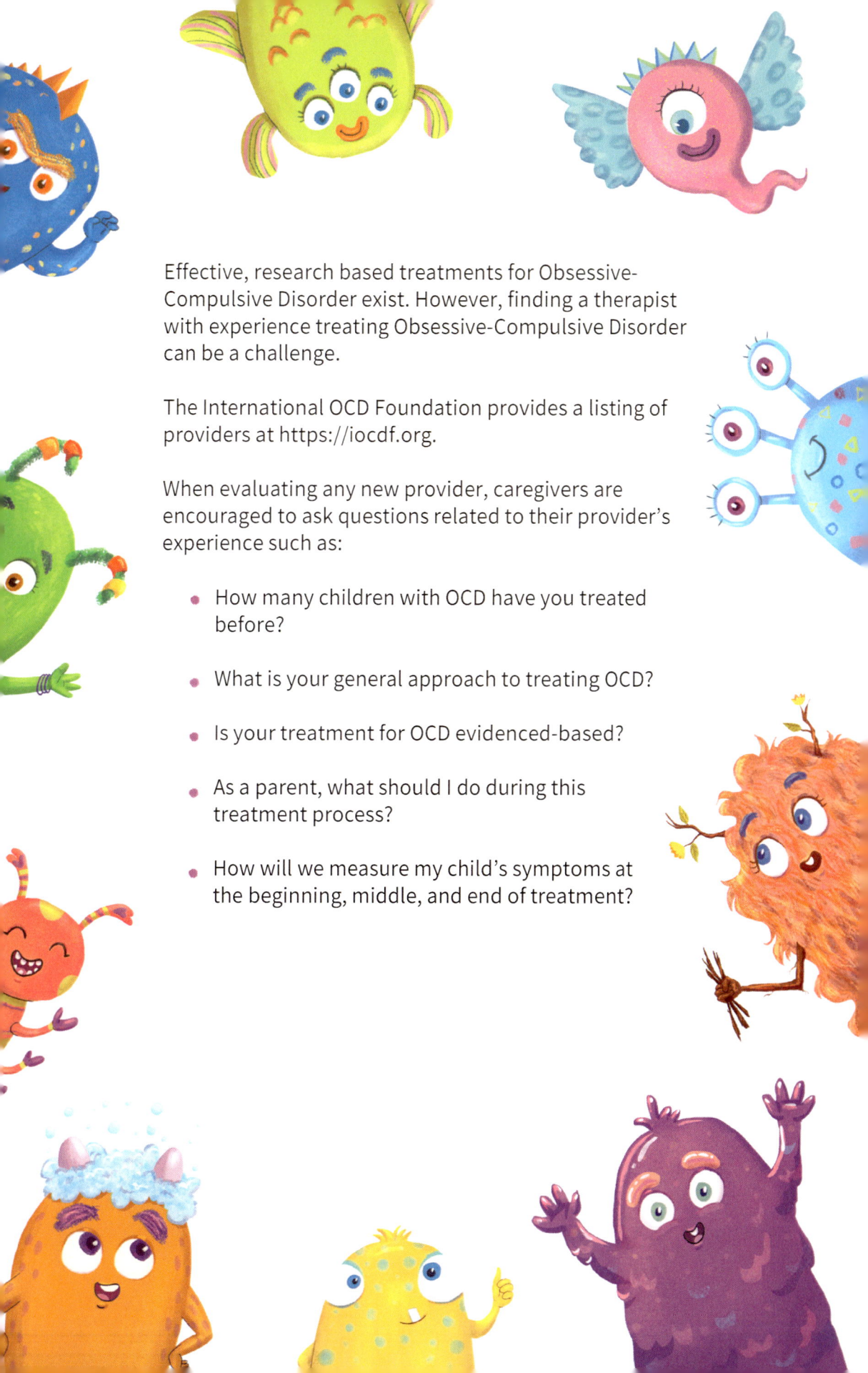

Effective, research based treatments for Obsessive-Compulsive Disorder exist. However, finding a therapist with experience treating Obsessive-Compulsive Disorder can be a challenge.

The International OCD Foundation provides a listing of providers at https://iocdf.org.

When evaluating any new provider, caregivers are encouraged to ask questions related to their provider's experience such as:

- How many children with OCD have you treated before?

- What is your general approach to treating OCD?

- Is your treatment for OCD evidenced-based?

- As a parent, what should I do during this treatment process?

- How will we measure my child's symptoms at the beginning, middle, and end of treatment?

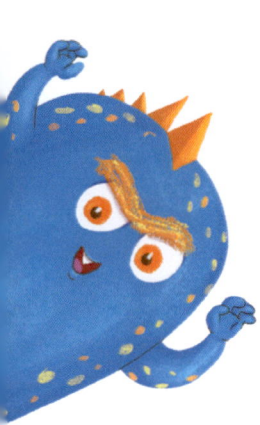

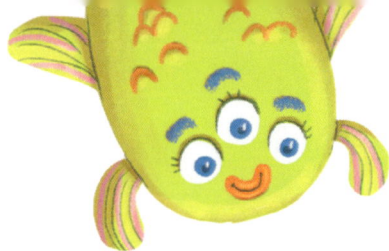

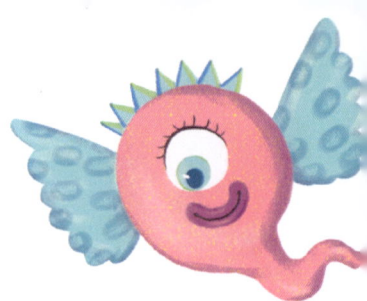

Now it's your turn!
In the space below, draw your Worry Monster.

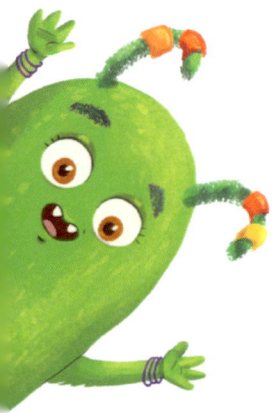

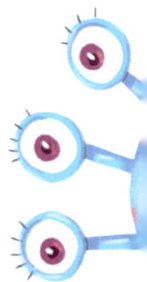

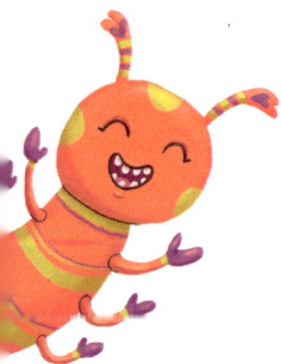

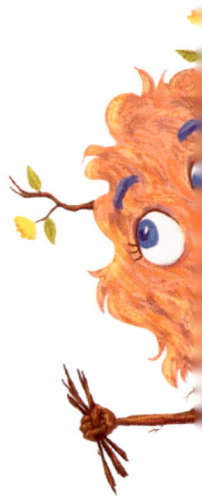

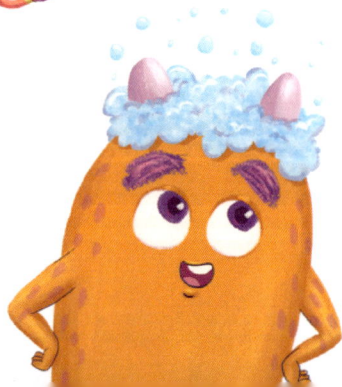

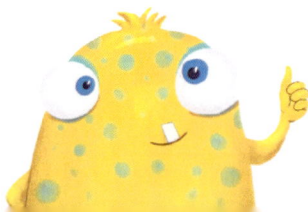

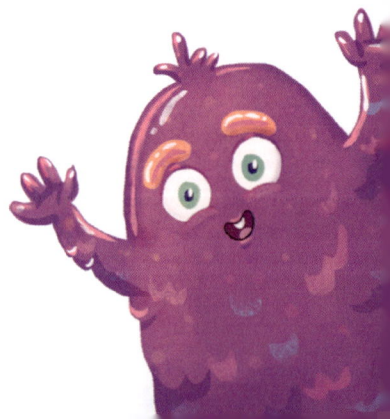

www.ingramcontent.com/pod-product-compliance
Lightning Source LLC
Chambersburg PA
CBRC101142030426
42335CB00008B/206